The Bach
Flower Remedies
Step by Step

The Bach
Flower Remedies
Step by Step

A complete guide to selecting
and using the remedies

BY JUDY RAMSELL HOWARD SRN, SCM, HV

*Fellow Custodian and Trustee
of The Bach Centre and the
Dr. E. Bach Healing Trust*

Vermilion
LONDON

This edition published in 2005 by Vermilion,
an imprint of Ebury Publishing

Ebury Publishing is a Random House Group company

First published in the United Kingdom in 1990 by
The C.W. Daniel Company Ltd

The Random House Group Limited Reg. No. 954009
www.randomhouse.co.uk

Addresses for companies within the Random House Group
can be found at www.randomhouse.co.uk

Penguin Random House is committed to a sustainable future for
our business, our readers and our planet. This book is made from
Forest Stewardship Council® certified paper.

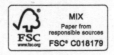

Printed and bound in Great Britain by Clays Ltd, St Ives plc

A CIP catalogue record for this book is available
from the British Library

ISBN: 9780091906535

Designed by Jane Norman

To buy books by your favourite authors and register for offers, visit
www.randomhouse.co.uk

Contents

My grateful thanks and dedication to:

My mother and father for their loving generosity;

My husband Keith for his support and patience;

My true friend Chris for her cheerful encouragement and inspiration for the title;

To George and Vina for their kindness and affection;

To all at the Bach Centre for their loyalty, especially my father for his enormous moral strength;

And to you the readers for taking an interest in Dr. Bach's work.

Further information, advice and details of supplies of remedies and books concerning the Bach Flower Remedies may be obtained from:

The Dr. Edward Bach Centre,
Mount Vernon,
Sotwell,
Wallingford,
Oxon. OX10 0PZ,
United Kingdom.
Tel: +44 (0)1491 834678

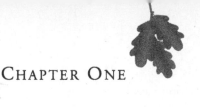

CHAPTER ONE

INTRODUCTION TO
DR. BACH'S HEALING REMEDIES

I can think of no better means of introducing the Bach Flower Remedies than to quote Dr. Bach's steadfast companion and devoted helper, Nora Weeks. Nora dedicated her life to the doctor's work, upholding all its principles and the most vital and fundamental essence of all, its simplicity. The following is an excerpt from a talk she gave many years ago. Dr. Bach's work is depicted beautifully by the person who knew it best.

"Will you, for the next half hour or so, turn your thoughts from the healing of the sick body to the healing of the sick person, for Dr. Edward Bach, after many years of research, gained the knowledge that our physical health depends upon our way of thinking, our feelings and emotions.

Good health is harmony, rhythm, when we think positively, constructively, happily. Ill-health when we think negatively, unhappily, destructively.

Such is the power of thought, the power man has over his body which is, after all, only the vehicle, the car he uses on his journey through life on earth.

As some of you may not know anything about the Bach Remedies, I would like first of all to tell you about Dr. Bach himself and how he developed this method of treatment and found the Flower Remedies.

The family came originally from Wales, so the name

should be 'Bach', but his medical colleagues always called him 'Batch', and we have done so ever since.

Edward Bach trained and qualified at University College Hospital and gained the Diploma of Public Health (D.P.H.) at Cambridge in the early 1900s. He was rather an unusual medical student, for he soon became more interested in the patients themselves than their diseases. He would sit by their bedsides and let them talk to him, and listening to them he found out the real cause of their ill-health. For instance, the woman with severe asthma was a very frightened woman. She told him her only son had taken a job in the north of England over three months ago and she had had no word from him in all that time. She was terrified that he had met with an accident, was badly injured, even that he had died. But one day he came to see her and told her he had found a job nearer home. Within a **few days** she lost her asthma completely. She no longer needed to hold her breath for her son.

The man with a suspected duodenal ulcer was a very worried man. He had lost his job, his wife was unable to work and he had two young children. Later, when he heard he had been reinstated in his work, he regained his health. He gained a job and lost his ulcer. The medical profession these days says that worry is often the cause of gastric and duodenal ulcers, but it was quite a new idea in those early days.

Dr. Bach began to feel then that treating the physical symptoms was not enough. The body was a mirror reflecting the thoughts in the mind. It was the sufferer himself, the person, who needed treatment and help to overcome his worries, fears, depressions, hopelessness. He felt that a completely new method of treatment was needed, a practical one, for words were not enough; it was of little use to say to a worried man, 'Don't worry, be happy'.

But first of all the doctor wanted to prove and test for himself other methods of orthodox medicines and he became a bacteriologist. He was well-known for his research work in this branch of medicine, but it did not satisfy him. He was still treating bodies and not people, and he much disliked the injection of the products of disease back into the human body. However, these years were not wasted, for he was studying his patients, his friends, everyone he came across, and watching their reactions to all the experiences of daily life; at work and at play, in good health and ill-health; and this knowledge of human nature was to stand him in good stead later on.

Then it was he came into contact with homoeopathy, and was delighted to find that Hahnemann, the founder of homoeopathy, had said, 'The patient is the most important factor in his healing'. Also, that homoeopathic remedies were prescribed for the personality of the patient, his characteristics, his idiosyncrasies as well as the physical symptoms.

Dr. Bach worked for some time in the laboratories of the Royal London Homoeopathic Hospital, and it was there that he became interested in the relationship between intestinal toxaemia and chronic disease. I want to tell you about this briefly, because the result of this research brought him a big step forward to his final work.

He isolated seven groups of intestinal flora and prepared nosodes from them homoeopathically, giving them to his patients by mouth. Their purpose is to cleanse and purify the intestinal tract. I say 'is', for these nosodes, the seven Bach nosodes, the seven bowel nosodes, are still being used today. They were most successful.

Then he made a most important and significant discovery. It was this: all the patients suffering from the same emotional difficulties needed the same nosode, irrespective of the type of physical disease. Those patients who were subject to violent emotional outbursts, brain storms, all needed the same nosode. Those who were nervous, apprehensive, again all needed another but the same nosode, no matter from what physical complaint they suffered.

From then onwards he prescribed these nosodes according to his patients' temperamental difficulties only. There was no need for a physical examination of the patient, laboratory tests were unnecessary and treatment could begin at once without delay. The results were excellent.

This confirmed his opinion that physical disease was not of physical origin, but that it was, as he said, 'the consolidation of a mental attitude'.

Dr. Bach now felt he could devote his time and his life to the search for the pure remedies which would help the sufferer rise above his unhappy thoughts. These new remedies he knew must be there for the finding in nature, amongst the trees and plants, for all our needs are provided for in nature by our Creator.

He already knew the principle of the new method of treatment: 'Treat the patient and not his disease', for when the negative thoughts had been overcome, the body would also respond.

So in 1930 he gave up all his work in London without a backward thought and went to live in the country.

Throughout all those years of medical practice he had been seeking for scientific proof of all his findings and using his intellect, but now a change occurred in himself. He became very sensitive both in mind and body.

Before finding a particular flower, he would suffer in himself and very acutely, the negative state of mind for which that flower was needed and, at the same time, he was privileged, as he said, to suffer from some physical complaint. Then he would wander about the fields and lanes until he found, or was led to find, the flower which would immediately restore his serenity and peace of mind, and within a few hours the physical complaint would also be healed.

In this way he found 38 flowers to cover the 38 negative states of mind from which mankind can suffer. These flowers, with three exceptions, are all the simple wild flowers of the countryside. He prepared the flowers only, for they grow above ground in the sunlight and the air and contain in their hearts the embryo seed, the continued life of the plant. You will know, of course, many of them – gorse, heather, honeysuckle, wild rose, chicory, agrimony – and the flowers of our well-known trees – oak, beech, willow, larch.

Dr. Bach placed the 38 remedies in seven groups. Those for fear; for uncertainty and indecision; for loneliness; for insufficient interest in present circumstances; for over-sensitiveness to ideas and influences; for despondency and despair; for over-care for the welfare of others.

In his little booklet 'The Twelve Healers & Other Remedies', he describes very simply the negative state of mind of each of these remedies."

Nora Weeks
1973

The full story of Dr. Bach's life can be read in "The Medical Discoveries of Edward Bach Physician" by Nora Weeks. It is a wonderful account of his career, research and eventual discovery of the healing properties of plants that have become so well-known throughout the world – the Bach Flower Remedies.

The 38 remedies constitute a complete system of healing; each plant having been specifically chosen for its primary function – the ability to treat the mind. Food plants and herbal remedies for other conditions have their own particular purpose, and so Dr. Bach bypassed these in his search for a clear and pure system of healing. Some people wonder whether he would have added more remedies had he lived longer, but he would not have done so because these 38 remedies provide for every negative state of mind and there can therefore be no others. And indeed, Dr. Bach declared his work complete shortly before he died in November 1936, and asked that it remain unaltered when he left its future in the hands of his dedicated helpers and companions. .

So although modern society challenges our lives with the pressures of its demanding pace, changing environment and "modern" diseases, human nature does not change, and although we may have to face different problems now to those in Dr. Bach's day, it is our emotional outlook which is important and that remains constant whatever the era might be. The fear of AIDS or cancer today is no different to the fear of diphtheria or smallpox prevalent during Dr. Bach's lifetime. The remedies treat the mental outlook, the personality trait and the temperament of the sufferer rather than the physical complaint directly, and so it is the fear which is important, not the smallpox or the AIDS. The remedies treat the person, not the disease, and although times change, the remedies move along with the people, not the time.

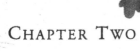

CHAPTER TWO

THE 38 REMEDIES

Dr. Bach intended the use of the remedies to be straightforward and simple enough for all to understand. He said:

> *"This work of healing has been done and published and given freely so that people like yourselves can help yourselves either in illness or to keep well and strong. It requires no science, only a little knowledge and sympathy and understanding of human nature, which is usual with almost all of us."*

Simplicity was his key-word and it was with this firmly uppermost in his mind that he wrote "The Twelve Healers & Other Remedies" which describes plainly and gently how each remedy is associated with various states of mind and outlook. That little booklet is the definitive text and is therefore the most essential of all books concerning the Bach Remedies.

Dr. Bach grouped the 38 remedies under seven headings:

1. For fear (Rock Rose, Mimulus, Cherry Plum, Aspen, Red Chestnut)

2. For uncertainty (Cerato, Scleranthus, Gentian, Gorse, Hornbeam, Wild Oat)

3. For insufficient interest in present circumstances (Clematis, Honeysuckle, Wild Rose, Olive, White Chestnut, Mustard, Chestnut Bud)

4. For loneliness (Water Violet, Impatiens, Heather)

5. For those over-sensitive to influence and ideas (Agrimony, Centaury, Walnut, Holly)

6. For despondency or despair (Larch, Pine, Elm, Sweet Chestnut, Star of Bethlehem, Willow, Oak, Crab Apple)

7. For over-care for welfare of others (Chicory, Vervain, Vine, Beech, Rock Water)

It is an important part of healing to be aware of why you are taking a remedy because this helps you to understand a little more about yourself and encourages you to be guided in a positive direction. The remedies are explained by describing the emotion or personality trait for which they are needed, but of course, there is a positive side to all of them. However, if the remedy becomes too aspirational, it may be so well disguised that it is difficult to appreciate what it is for. Therefore I have tried to offer balanced, straightforward descriptions because I believe everyone can relate to emotions they know and understand. For easy reference, the remedies appear in alphabetical order.

AGRIMONY

This remedy is for those who hide their feelings behind a brave and cheerful face. They are normally bright and happy people, often vivacious, and others rarely see the anxiety which may be harboured within. Pain, worry, ill-health are swept aside with a light breezy remark, pretending all is well. Their inner suffering can be torture for them at times, but they still try to maintain a smile so that their feelings remain hidden. But keeping the mask in place only adds to their burden. The Agrimony remedy helps those of this nature when they are in distress to relax within themselves so that they can put their difficulties into perspective and share their problems if necessary.

ASPEN

The Aspen has often been referred to as "the trembling tree" because its leaves appear to shiver and whisper in the breeze. This is quite apt because the Aspen remedy is one for fear. Not fear of known things – the remedy for that is Mimulus – but for the unknown fears which can be quite disturbing and fill the sufferer with panic for no apparent reason. The Aspen fear takes the form of apprehension, anxious anticipation, foreboding or dread. But when the sufferer is asked what he or she is afraid of, nothing specific can be identified and they cannot explain why they are so fearful.

BEECH

Those who require this remedy find it difficult to understand the shortcomings of others. Beech people can be very critical of the behaviour of those whom they consider foolish, shortsighted or ignorant and therefore often lack tolerance and empathy. They find people's habits and idiosyncrasies annoying and although they consider themselves to be perfectionists, they find it difficult to appreciate that others too have their own set of ideals and therefore might have good reason to act the way they do. Beech people are not necessarily forthright – in many ways they can appear to be quite patient and calm, yet are often seething with irritation inside! The Beech remedy helps those of this nature to step for a moment into another's shoes in order to adopt a more understanding and tolerant attitude.

CENTAURY

This is the remedy which gives strength to those who find it hard to stand up for themselves. They are full of kindness and are ever-willing, always eager to help or be of service. It goes against their nature to say "no" as they do not like to let anyone down, and because of their gentle and generous nature, they are easily dominated or manipulated and often find themselves the victim of stronger, more powerful personalities who may take advantage of their kind-heartedness. The Centaury person may then become exhausted by over-work and begin to despise him or herself for being so weak. The remedy helps these gentle folk to remain gentle but firm when the need arises so that they gain more respect and appreciation.

Dr. Bach described the Centaury character beautifully in a little story:

> *"I am weak, yes, I know I am weak, but why? Because I have learnt to hate strength and power and dominion, and if I do err a little on the weakness side, forgive me, because it is only a reaction to the hatred of hurting others, and I shall soon learn to understand how to find the balance when I neither hurt nor am hurting. But just for the moment I would rather that I suffered than that I caused one moment's pain to my brother."*

CERATO

This remedy is for those who distrust their own judgement. When they make a decision they question it and often ask the advice or opinion of others as a form of reassurance and confirmation. Alas, these people can be swayed by the thoughts and ideas of those whose opinions they seek and as a result may take the wrong path. Then they say, "I KNEW I should have done so and so". Or they might ask the advice of every friend, asking "What shall I do?", "What would you do if you were me?", and then, having absorbed all the answers, decide to do it their own way after all! Ceratos waste so much time through their dilemma that they can miss out on many opportunities. This differs from the indecision of Scleranthus people, however, because the latter do not usually voice their uncertainty, whereas Cerato types need to draw on the opinions of others to give clarity to their own thoughts. They also differ from Larch people because although Cerato folk lack confidence in their judgement, once they have made up their mind, they do have the confidence to take up the challenge and often succeed. The Larch person would rather stand back and let the opportunity pass them by, feeling far too self-conscious to make any attempt.

CHERRY PLUM

This remedy is for the desperate fear of the mind giving way, of insanity and of the impulse to do harm to other people or to oneself. It is therefore the remedy for those who become prone to thoughts of suicide. The Cherry Plum state may follow a long period of anxiety or depression and those in this desperate frame of mind are often on the verge of a nervous breakdown or feel that they are on the point of madness. The remedy can, however, also be of help when the mood is of an acute or sudden nature, and is indicated wherever there is lack of emotional control such as sudden outbursts of irrational and sometimes uncharacteristic rage or violence or hysteria, and for this reason is included in the Rescue Remedy (see page 37).

CHESTNUT BUD

The sticky ripening bud of the Horse Chestnut is the remedy to help those who cannot learn the lessons of life. When confronted with a situation for the second or third time, these people do not draw on their experience of the first incident and so find themselves repeating the same mistake, sometimes time and time again.

Chestnut Bud helps such people to observe the lessons of each experience so that they do not suffer the distress of repeated mistakes.

CHICORY

Chicory is the remedy for those who are of a "mothering" type. They are loving and kind but have a tendency to fuss and are therefore inclined to be over-protective. They are happiest when they feel needed, with their family around them to organize and manage. This loving concern, however, can become overpowering at times causing those they care for to feel stifled by such a strong emotional embrace. They then attempt to hold on to their loved ones, becoming selfish and possessive, feeling rejected and easily hurt, and adopting a "no-one appreciates me" attitude. The Chicory remedy helps these people to let go, to love and advise without demanding love and attention in return. It is also helpful for children who "cling" and demand constant attention, and who become possessive over friends or toys.

CLEMATIS

Those of the Clematis type are often of a creative, artistic nature and love to have something to look forward to; something to fantasize about. They can therefore lack interest in the present because their minds are full of hopes and dreams of the future. They may become inattentive, dreamy and absent minded and appear to be in a world of their own, oblivious of what is going on around them. They are inclined to lack concentration and easily become bored with a conversation or event which is not dynamic enough to hold their interest. It may be said of the Clematis type that they hear without listening, see without looking, and forget what they are saying or what is being said to them. This remedy is indicated whenever this state of mind is apparent and is also helpful where there is mental escapism, especially into a sleepy dream-world (like the dormouse from Alice in Wonderland!). It is therefore helpful where consciousness is lost, fainting or where there is a sensation of faintness or bemused state of mind, and for these reasons is included in the Rescue Remedy (see page 37).

CRAB APPLE

This is known as the "cleansing remedy" and is indicated whenever there is a feeling of having been soiled, for example by disease, pollution, touching a dirty object or dealing with infected material. In such instances, there is an intense feeling of uncleanliness and a compulsion to rid the system of the "poison". On occasions, this urge is so great that those in need of this remedy feel they must wash over and over again because they are convinced they have been contaminated in some way. They can be very houseproud and quite fastidious with regard to hygiene generally, closely inspecting their knife and fork in a restaurant before eating their meal, for example.

Crab Apple is also indicated where there is a feeling of self-disgust or self-loathing, when the reflection of oneself in a mirror causes repulsion; and for those revolted by such things as food and eating, bodily functions, sex or sickness.

Another aspect of this remedy is in the help it gives to those whose minds are full of trivial details to the exclusion of more important ones. Nora Weeks gave the example of the brave woman who was far more concerned about the psoriasis on her elbows than the inoperable cancer from which she was suffering. This remedy helps such people to see things in their true proportion. Dr. Bach described it as "the remedy which helps us to get rid of anything we do not like either in our minds or our bodies".

ELM

Elm is the remedy for those who, at times, find that the pressures and responsibility of their work or family commitments become overwhelming, leaving them feeling inadequate and worn out. They are usually capable people and may indeed hold a responsible position, but when the burden of their responsibility, whatever it might be, begins to pile up, it eventually becomes too heavy to bear. The Elm state can, under such circumstances, give way to panic at not being able to cope, and those who suffer this way feel they cannot take any more. This can be especially stressful if the person concerned holds a position of importance, when their capability and competence is crucial, or is a person upon whom others rely. The remedy helps the mind to become calmer so that the problem can be put into perspective and thought about clearly, rationally and methodically, thus encouraging the confidence, which has been temporarily lost, to return.

GENTIAN

This remedy is for despondency and discouragement, occurring as a result of a disappointment, for example failing an examination or interview, losing a job, and other events or set-backs which make one feel depressed. Gentian is also helpful when the mind fills with doubt of one's ability to succeed after an initial failure, when one is then inclined to lose faith. The Gentian remedy lifts the spirits and gives the encouragement needed to persevere or try again. It helps to dispel negative thinking and allows a positive attitude to return so that instead of sinking into a well of self-doubt and heavy-heartedness, one's approach to the particular challenge which lies ahead, whatever it might be, becomes much more optimistic. "I will succeed" is the Gentian motto!

GORSE

If the Gentian despondency is "nipped in the bud" and appropriately treated, the hopelessness of the Gorse state will be prevented. But sometimes the transition from one to the other takes place so quickly that the Gorse state of mind can take hold with little warning. The discouragement soon develops into despair and the sufferer becomes so forlorn that he or she is filled with utter hopelessness. A second attempt after a disappointing failure seems useless and the Gorse person will not try again. When ill, these people do not expect good health to return and they give up hope of ever getting better. If help is sought, it is often due to the persuasion of a friend, but the Gorse person is so pessimistic that he or she has no hope of the treatment working. They might say, "Well I'll try if you want me to, but I don't suppose it will do me any good. Nothing can help so there's little point in bothering". If these people do, however, give their remedy a chance, hope will begin to return and this will lift them out of their gloom and help them to realise that all their prospects and chances are not lost.

HEATHER

Heather people are chatterboxes! Dr. Bach fondly named them "buttonholers" because they like to come close to you and talk into your face. They also like to touch you, nudge you, or hold your arm to keep your attention. They enjoy talking about themselves, their family and friends and when unwell will talk of nothing but their ailments. Their audience has difficulty contributing to the conversation and even when they do, it merely serves to feed the Heather person with a cue or reminder to tell yet another story about themselves! They dislike being alone and are unhappy and depleted when they are, for they live on the vitality of others, sap their strength and leave them exhausted. For this reason other people tend to avoid them and they become lonely as a result. Nora Weeks described a man in the village who was of this type ... "if he saw you coming he would get off his bicycle, prop it against the hedge and settle down for a long chat. He would tell you of his catarrh, his varicose veins, his indigestion and, if you tried to move away, he would grip you by the arm and say 'but I must tell you this ...'. Eventually he came to ask for treatment for a rash on his hands. He was given Heather of course, and he gradually began to take an interest in other people, listening to them instead of talking about himself. People began to like him, and his rash disappeared."

Another indication for Heather is when there is total self-absorption or obsession with one's troubles or ailments; when the mind thinks of nothing else. The remedy then helps the sufferer to take their mind off themselves and so consider the other important issues of life going on around them.

HOLLY

This remedy is for jealousy, envy, hatred, revenge, suspicion. The emotion is strong and burning and can give rise to outbursts of temper. Similar feelings which create a more inward, sulky resentment are dealt with by Willow (page 36), whereas Holly is for the more explosive feelings. Depending on the personality concerned, these feelings may or may not be outwardly revealed. Some people will keep their feelings to themselves, in others their temper will flare, which might require the addition of Cherry Plum if there is a lack of emotional control and fear of becoming violent. Holly emotions can also cause a great deal of anger, but "anger" is a word which can describe many states of mind such as frustration (Vervain), aggression (Vine), intolerance (Beech), impatience (Impatiens), and so it is necessary to consider the causes and reasons for the anger to determine whether Holly is in fact the most appropriate remedy.

HONEYSUCKLE

Those who are in this frame of mind miss much of life because they are pre-occupied with the events of the past, whether these be happy or sad. They dwell on memories of life gone by, thoughts of their childhood, homesickness, regrets of past mistakes or missed opportunities, and they spend their time sentimentally reminiscing about "the good old days", wishing things could be as they were or had been different. "If only" is frequently uttered by those in need of this remedy. The state of mind can soon develop into a loss of interest in the issues and demands of today. You will remember the mental escapism of the Clematis folk who dream of the future – Honeysuckle people retreat into the past.

The remedy can help those who have suffered a bereavement (in addition to Star of Bethlehem for the shock, sorrow and grief – see page 31), when the mind is full of memories surrounding the person they have lost. Honeysuckle helps such people to remember and reflect on past happiness and cherish their memories without losing sight of the importance of their own present existence. It helps them take that necessary step forward.

Sometimes past memories are unpleasant and disturbing and may haunt a person's mind with a vivid recollection of an unhappy or traumatic experience. This may have repercussions during sleep and cause repeated dreams or nightmares (see also Rock Rose for terror – page 29).

Honeysuckle helps to focus the mind on the present and puts the past into perspective, allowing us to draw on it for experience and to recall momentarily some pleasant or loving memory, without it dominating our thoughts.

HORNBEAM

This remedy gives emotional strength to those who cannot face the day ahead or cannot enthuse about some project or duty to which they should attend. It is not due to exhaustion or tiredness from overwork – this requires the Olive remedy (page 27) – but is rather a mental weariness at the thought of what lies ahead. It causes procrastination and lethargy so that work which was once a pleasure becomes a chore. It is, however, rather like the familiar "Monday morning feeling", and once work has begun and the day's routine is in progress, the feeling disappears.

IMPATIENS

Impatiens, as the name suggests, is for the state of impatience and irritability. Those of this temperament tend to be quick in thought and action. Everything is done in a hurry; they cannot wait. People with this nature can become quite brusque with those who are slow and may be tempted to finish a sentence for them, or try to finish the job they are doing. Impatiens people tend to be restless, fretful and jumpy. They move and talk quickly and their body language too can give them away – fidgeting, looking at their watch, edging towards the door in their haste. The remedy simply helps these people to regain their poise so that life is not so rushed; so that they may take their time and enjoy the pleasure of life at a normal pace.

The remedy is indicated whenever there is irritability or restlessness due to impatience, and although there is an Impatiens "type" as described above, the remedy will benefit people of any personality if this frame of mind is prevalent. It is included in the Rescue Remedy for its calming effect when the trauma has caused a degree of mental agitation.

LARCH

The red flowers of the sweeping branches of the larch are to help those who lack confidence in themselves. Larch is for the kind of people who, although they may have the ability or capability, do not believe it of themselves and so they stand back in the shadows allowing others to take their place. Consequently, many of life's opportunities pass them by because of their lack of self-reliance. If an opportunity comes their way they are inclined to say, "I wouldn't possibly be able to do that", full of doubt about their own ability and afraid of failure. This contrasts with the Cerato personalities who have faith in their ability to carry out a certain task, but so doubt their judgement that they delay and often do not carry it through.

Dr. Bach said, "Let us plunge into life. We are here to gain experience and knowledge, and we shall learn but little unless we face realities and seek to our utmost". The Larch remedy helps those who do not have sufficient confidence, to be a little bolder so that they too can plunge into life.

MIMULUS

This is the remedy for fear of known things – fear of illness, poverty, living alone, travelling, of death or injury – the fears of everyday life. The remedy will help people, whatever their personality, if they are afraid, but there is a side to Mimulus which describes a certain type of person. Those of the Mimulus nature are often afraid of people and are shy, nervous or retiring. They feel uneasy with people they do not know and tend to blush easily or stammer in their presence. They therefore dislike social gatherings because they feel too self conscious to join in, and feel intimidated by the exuberance of others. The Mimulus remedy helps these timid, bashful folk to have the courage to confront their fears, and as they do, so their fears diminish, just as a dark room ceases to be frightening once the light has been switched on.

MUSTARD

Mustard is the remedy for the kind of depression which descends like a dark cloud and hides the sunshine and joy of life. The mood then sinks into a melancholic misery, the heart feeling like a lead weight. People who suffer from the Mustard state are very unhappy but when asked why they feel that way, they cannot find a reason. They will often say that they have everything they want: a loving family, a comfortable home, holidays, no financial worries, yet they feel so low, and cannot understand why. But the Mustard depression never has a cause. The mood descends for no apparent reason and may remain for days, weeks or even months, until it eventually lifts as suddenly as it came, only to return again and again in a fluctuating cycle. The Mustard remedy helps to dispel the dark cloud which overshadows the life of these people, and thus allows the sunshine to fill their lives once again.

OAK

There is very little which is negative about the Oak temperament – these people are the fighters, they do not give up hope or give in to adversity. They are solid and reliable, just like the Oak tree itself, and others often go to the Oak for guidance or comfort. When ill or incapacitated, the Oaks will struggle on regardless, despite their body's call for rest, considering such restrictions to be a hindrance. They are the type to simply roll up their sleeves and get on with it! But sometimes, these people can overdo things and because they have ignored the alarm signals of tiredness or pain, they eventually find their strength is no longer there. This causes them to feel unhappy and annoyed with themselves and it is then that they need their Oak remedy to help them rebuild their strength.

OLIVE

This remedy is for exhaustion, sufferers being so drained of energy that they feel too tired to go on. The Olive weariness differs from that of Hornbeam because Olive people are fatigued due to overwork or over-exertion. Hornbeam people cannot find the enthusiasm to even begin their work. Once depleted of their strength in this way, life itself becomes hard work for the Olive folk and eventually ceases to be enjoyable. When this state occurs,

Olive helps to revivify and replenish lost energy. The remedy is also helpful for those studying for examinations and for those involved with intricate or heavy mental work, as well as those who are physically exhausted. It is also recommended following illness when the person is weak and tired.

PINE

The Pine remedy is for feelings of guilt. This may stem from the past, the sufferer harbouring their guilt for many years, or it may be due to something more recent. Those who need this remedy frequently are those who blame themselves even for the mistakes of others, and are always apologizing. They are full of remorse and burden themselves with self-reproach even when they have done no wrong.

RED CHESTNUT

This remedy is to help those who are afraid of something happening to their loved ones. It is only natural to be apprehensive when children are away from home for the first time, or if your partner has to travel a long distance, but for the Red Chestnut people, this fear is out of all proportion in their minds and they become desperately afraid that some disaster will occur, that their children will catch pneumonia if they are not kept warm or that their partner will be involved in an accident, and they will not rest until their loved ones are safely home again. These people do not worry about themselves – their only concern is for the health and safety of their family. Their love does not become selfish or possessive like the Chicory folk, but because they are so afraid and so worried, they tend to fuss and fret which, like the Chicory type, can make their loved ones feel overwhelmed by their concern, and this may instil similar fears in their children and so deplete their natural confidence. The Red Chestnut remedy helps these people to put their fears into perspective so that they can love and care for their family without losing sight of rational thought or the reality of the situation.

ROCK ROSE

This is the remedy for extreme fear; terror, panic. It may not always be rational, but is nevertheless very real. Those who suffer from this state of mind are truly scared and as a result may tremble or perspire with fright. This awful fear may be the result of a horrifying accident, causing the person to become terrified of travelling, undergoing a serious operation, hospitalisation and so on. Rock Rose would be indicated in all these circumstances and would also help both children and adults who are troubled by nightmares. Do not confuse it with the description of Mimulus, the remedy for all known fears. If the fear creates panic or sheer terror, then Rock Rose would always be the more appropriate remedy.

ROCK WATER

Those of this nature are so strict with themselves that they may live by a rigid regime or set of standards. They may be very religious or have certain other ideals which govern their lives, and as they strive to achieve these ideals or follow their particular faith, they chastise themselves if they should stray from their determined path. They expect perfection in all they do and dislike shoddiness, laziness or a similar attitude in others. They do not, however, openly criticize peoples' shortcomings, but play the martyr, showing their disapproval by setting an example for others to follow. They are self-righteous and generally proudly enjoy their stringent lifestyle. They would need their remedy if, as is often the case, their high standards become so harsh and inflexible that they deny themselves even the simplest pleasures in life. This can lead to much tension, self-reproach and unhappiness, and the Rock Water remedy helps these people to be less rigid and more lenient with themselves.

SCLERANTHUS

This little plant helps those who suffer emotional distress through indecision. These people have difficulty in choosing between two things and it is a problem for them in everyday situations as well as where more important decisions are concerned. A dilemma arises whenever a choice has to be made. When out shopping they might see two shirts they like, and spend much time looking at one and then the other, trying to decide which they prefer. Even when eventually a choice is made, there is still doubt. They may hesitate at the cash-desk, turning away and replacing the shirt on the rail, only to return five minutes later having decided to buy it after all. This "ping-pong" state of mind causes these people mental trauma. They do not, however, usually discuss their difficulties with others as would the Cerato person. They struggle with their uncertainty alone and it can become tiring and create much mental agitation. The Scleranthus remedy helps these people to bring their thoughts into focus so that they can see the options more clearly and learn to know their own minds.

Other indications for this remedy include mood swings, fluctuations between happiness and tears; gentleness and anger and so on – whenever there is a rapid change of mood. The remedy is helpful whenever there is an imbalance of this nature, the mind not knowing which direction to take. It can therefore be of help for motion or travel sickness when the unsteadiness of the vehicle is disturbing.

STAR OF BETHLEHEM

This is Dr. Bach's remedy for shock and is indicated whenever there has been trauma to the system, for example through accident, disturbing news, or a distressing sight. Following a bereavement it helps the bereaved to cope with their grief and ease their pain and sorrow. Sometimes the shock of losing someone dear cannot be expressed; the person at times longing to cry but tears will not come. Star of Bethlehem helps to unblock this passage and relieves the mind of its sadness.

Shock can be delayed, and may eventually manifest itself in a number of ways, sometimes many years after the event. But even if treatment is sought for some other difficulty, if shock has been sustained and can be identified as the cause of the trouble, Star of Bethlehem should always be included. If the shock can be treated without delay, however, the impact of the trauma is lessened and for this reason it is one of the five remedies Dr. Bach included in the Rescue Remedy.

SWEET CHESTNUT

This remedy is for a desperate mental anguish; a feeling of utter despair as though there is no light at the end of the tunnel. Those suffering this way feel that there is nothing left in life and are so sad that they may physically hurt inside, feeling desolate and heartbroken. They feel so wretched that at times they may wish they could die, but are not usually inclined towards suicide because they do not believe even death will release them from their pain. They can see no way out of their inner darkness and life holds no joy for them. The Sweet Chestnut remedy helps to raise the curtain of despair so that faith is restored. The horizon becomes brighter and hope returns to their lives; the end of the torment at last within reach.

VERVAIN

Those of this nature have strong principles and ethics, and when faced with a situation which goes against their ideals, they feel they must put their point of view forward. In so doing, they try to convince and convert others to their way of thinking. Like the Rock Water types, they too are perfectionists but are more concerned for the welfare and growth of others, usually the underdog or under-privileged, than motivated by self-interest as are Rock Water people. Vervain folk tend to feel strongly about matters such as the environment, politics, religion, world famine, housing and poverty, their feelings often strong enough to initiate the formation of pressure groups, and will often write to their MP, attend meetings and so on. This, however, is their release, and if they are unable to find an outlet for their vehemence, they become frustrated and tense. Vervain people tend to be active, always on the go; involving themselves in several jobs at once, their minds racing ahead to what should be done next. They enjoy a challenge and are enthusiastic about their aims, but because of their nature, they can push themselves so hard that they are unable to relax and feel in a state of tension as though they are living with the elastic stretched. The Vervain remedy helps them to wind down so that they can relax and give themselves a chance to rest.

VINE

Vine is the remedy for those who are self-assured, dominant, the leaders and rulers. They know their own minds absolutely, making decisions and taking responsibility, for themselves as well as others, without hesitation. Vine people are ambitious and determined, tackling life's problems with confidence and certainty. In a team they take the leading role, directing others with incontestable frankness. They will say, "THIS is what you will do", rather than "Would you like to do it this way?" or "Shall we do this?" Like the Vervain, Vine people have fixed opinions, but whereas the Vervain would try to convince others that they are right through explanation or debate, the Vine person would not argue the matter. He or she would make their point and that would be that. In the extreme, the Vine nature can be demanding and powerful, and those in subservient positions may become emotionally crippled as a result if they themselves do not have sufficient strength of character to stand up to (what can be) a tyrannical Vine. The gentle and ever willing Centaury person is often a victim!

Children of the Vine nature are demanding, aggressive, take charge of peer groups, and in the extreme can become bullies to those of a weaker or more gentle nature.

The Vine remedy does not take this self-assurance or leadership away, for indeed these are fine and positive qualities to have, but when the extreme side of the nature takes an upper hand, the remedy will help these people to be less harsh and severe, and more understanding of the views of others and the plight of those who are weaker.

WALNUT

Walnut is the remedy for change. It helps those who have difficulty settling into a new environment, new job or routine, a different country or new home. It helps to break the link with the past so that life can start afresh, free from old ties and memories. It is helpful during any change in life, from marriage, divorce or moving house to the major growth milestones of teething, puberty and menopause, and can help with the adjustment to childbirth and to the changes during the menstrual cycle.

The remedy also helps us to keep to our chosen path in life, protecting us from the ideas and influences of others that may lead us astray, and from those disturbing environmental influences which disrupt our peace and taunt our thoughts, and which may cause us to lose sight of our true destination. Those who need the Walnut remedy are often sensitive people who are easily disturbed by such disruptive influences. The remedy helps to guide us through these events in life so that we do not lose our way.

WATER VIOLET

As with Oak and Vine, the Water Violet nature is a very positive one. These people, like the plant itself, stand proud and erect. They prefer the quieter things in life and for this reason tend to be reserved. They move about quietly, are not clumsy or erratic but serene and self-assured. They are not gregarious people and find their own company or that of a few well chosen friends more harmonious than large social gatherings. Their outlook is one of superiority and they like to keep themselves to themselves. They are willing to give advice if requested, but do not attempt to interfere or influence, and similarly will not discuss their own health or concerns with others. They therefore suffer and bear their grief in silence and because they keep a thin veil between themselves and those around them, they tend to distance themselves from people. The thin veil can become a hard barrier which is difficult to penetrate and the Water Violet then finds that people are in awe of them, find them remote and unapproachable, supercilious or condescending and this can cause them much loneliness. The remedy helps to break down this barrier and thus enables them to welcome others with friendliness and yet retain their calm serenity, and to remain proud without appearing haughty.

WHITE CHESTNUT

This remedy is indicated whenever the mind is tormented by worrying or repetitive and unwanted thoughts. Dr. Bach called this the "gramaphone record remedy" because these persistent thoughts, mental arguments or conversations go round and round in the mind like a long playing record and are so difficult to stop that they leave the sufferer exhausted and unable to concentrate. The White Chestnut remedy helps to relieve this mental whirlpool and restore peace of mind.

WILD OAT

This remedy is for those who feel they have come to a cross-roads in life and do not know which way to go. They want to do something fulfilling but are not certain in which direction they should channel their energies. They may have tried several careers or a variety of lifestyles but still do not feel content. They are the "lost souls" who feel they have not yet found their niche in life and are filled with dissatisfaction. This remedy helps these people to see the way ahead more clearly so that they may pursue their true vocation.

The Wild Oat person differs from the Scleranthus because the latter always finds decisions difficult to make, and debates even the most trivial of matters. The Wild Oat people, however, are filled with uncertainty when they reach a "cross-roads" in their lives, but are otherwise decisive, determined and clear in their thoughts.

WILD ROSE

Unlike Wild Oat, Wild Rose people do not have the enthusiasm or ambition to change anything in life and therefore drift along without effort or motivation. They are inclined to become apathetic and resigned to all that happens, quietly accepting whatever lies in store for them. If misfortune occurs they will say, "Oh well, that's life". Wild Rose people are "happy as they are", do not like change and may therefore pass up many opportunities because too much effort is required of them. They are passive people and easily surrender to the struggle of life. If they become ill they will give in to their illness and if this should cause some disability will meekly submit to "having to live with it". The Wild Rose state can be one of emotional flatness, feeling neither happy nor sad, excited nor depressed, and can therefore lack vital energy and sparkle. The Wild Rose remedy helps these people to revive their inner zest for life so that although they will remain happy to sail along on the current of life, they do so with contented awareness instead of disinterest.

WILLOW

This remedy is for those whose thoughts have become so introspective that they dwell on their misfortune. They feel resentful that life has treated them so badly, wondering what they have done to deserve such hardship. They become wrapped up in self-pity, grumble, moan or sulk and, when things go wrong, find it hard to look on the bright side and forgive and forget. When adversity strikes, they turn it inwards upon themselves where it festers away creating a big "chip on the shoulder" and generating an attitude of "Poor old me, nobody cares!" They feel very hard done by and bitter, and blame others for their unhappy state. They feel sorry for themselves and find it hard to be cheerful because "there is nothing to be cheerful about", and can only see things from a negative angle. They forget that there is a positive side to every situation. The Willow remedy therefore helps to lift the sufferer out of this hollow of self-mortification so that he or she may adopt a more optimistic and positive approach to life.

THE COMPOSITE RESCUE REMEDY

There is one other remedy which is frequently needed. It contains five of the 38 remedies and is called Rescue Remedy. As the name suggests, it is the remedy for all emergencies and is therefore indicated whenever an emergency situation arises in which there is panic, shock, mental numbness etc. Obviously it does not take the place of medical attention but as it helps to alleviate the mental anguish, it enables the body's own healing processes to begin without delay. Rescue Remedy is also very calming in other traumatic situations such as flying, visiting the dentist, taking an examination or before an important interview.

Rescue Remedy can be taken orally and applied externally if necessary (to stings, sprains, bruises etc) and is available both in liquid form and as a cream (see Ch. 4, page 71 for methods of administration).

Animals can also benefit from the remedies and in

particular Rescue Remedy because there is nearly always an element of shock or terror associated with or responsible for an animal's discomfort. Plants too respond very well and many have revived after a few drops of Rescue Remedy! (see page 62).

The five remedies which are combined together to form the Rescue Remedy are:

STAR OF BETHLEHEM – for shock

ROCK ROSE – for great fear and panic

IMPATIENS – for mental and physical tension when the sufferer cannot relax; the mind agitated and irritable

CHERRY PLUM – for loss of emotional control, when the sufferer screams, shouts or becomes hysterical

CLEMATIS – the remedy for the bemused, distant feeling which often precedes a faint

These five remedies were specifically chosen by Dr. Bach as an emergency composite because combined they form an appropriate all-round crisis remedy. He first used Rescue Remedy in the early 1930s when he gave it to a fisherman who had only just survived a shipwreck. The young fisherman was unconscious and blue in the face. As he was carried up the beach, Dr. Bach moistened his lips, behind his ears and wrists with the remedy. He soon regained consciousness and, as though awakening from a bad dream, sat up and asked for a cigarette.

CHAPTER THREE

REMEDY SELECTION

Understanding the Bach System

It is emphasised throughout the Bach Remedy literature that the treatment is based on personality, and so whatever the problem might be, the remedies should be selected according to the emotional outlook, the mood, temperament and personality of the individual concerned.

Dr. Bach strongly believed that physical ill-health was a result of a disequilibrium within our minds and that it was therefore of utmost importance to treat the mind in order to bring about healing of the sick body. Indeed, there are many instances where this philosophy is well established and accepted within medicine generally. Tension, anxiety, worry and so on all have the potential to create a variety of physical problems, manifesting in different ways. We have all experienced the feeling of "butterflies" when nervous or excited, or been aware of a dryness in the mouth, clammy, trembling hands or a thumping in the chest when afraid or apprehensive. These are all physical sensations, not imaginary but very real, and yet they all occur as a result of an emotional disturbance. These reactions, however, are generally relatively short lasting and usually occur prior to a certain given situation such as an examination or driving test, meeting someone for the first time, speaking in public, going to hospital or visiting the dentist. If these occasions can have such a profound impact on our physical being, then it follows that a prolonged emotional struggle will have an even greater impact. Our body will only be able to cope with a certain amount of strain before it begins to protest and eventually starts to break down. We all have our "weak spots" and may therefore suffer in different ways. For some, stress and strain may result in migraine, for others asthma, for others digestive problems or skin disorders, and although the person may have always felt this weakness to be present, fear or worry or anxiety often initiates an attack or causes an acute worsening of the condition. In effect, this is the body's built-in safety mechanism and acts as a warning signal telling us that we are pushing ourselves too hard, that we should take time to recuperate and rest. However, the pressures of life are such that it is not always possible to take a rest on demand, or stop our work when we want to. Others may depend on us and so we keep going ... Eventually something has to give way, and just like a motorcar, the body's "exhaust" must either dissipate or be released. If the physical constitution is strong, an emotional breakdown may occur. But whatever the result, it is the cause that matters.

There are, however, certain conditions which do not have a definite emotional cause. Let us again consider asthma and migraine as examples. We have discussed how these may be caused or made worse by emotional upset, but sometimes it is the case that these and certain other conditions, are found to be the result of an allergic reaction to a particular food or environmental irritant. Migraine, for example, is often associated with eating cheese or chocolate; asthma with house dust or cat fur. Hay fever is another example and is, as we know, exacerbated by pollen or certain grasses. However, not everyone who is exposed to pollen suffers with hay fever; similarly, many people live with animals with no ill-effects.

We therefore have to ask why it is that some people are particularly sensitive and suffer such a reaction. To address this problem fully, we need to consider the person as a whole, taking into account their personality, lifestyle and associated emotional influences. It is only then that the TRUE cause of their problem can be approached and complete treatment achieved.

There are some conditions of course, which are, however, purely organic in origin, and although the Bach Remedies have an important role to play in re-establishing the person's overall well-being, a more conventional, orthodox approach may be essential. A burst appendix for example requires immediate medical attention, as would severe intestinal blockage or a broken limb. Similarly, if we take a poison it will make us very ill – we are only human after all! The remedies, therefore, cannot take the place of vital medical treatment when it is needed and it should always be sought if there is any doubt or cause for concern about your physical health.

However, whatever the problem, there is no doubt that worry, fear, depression, self-pity and other negative emotions which so often accompany ill-health, hinder our recovery and retard convalescence. But because the remedies treat these negative feelings, with their help our inner strength can be revived and this will aid our recovery and return to health.

Learning to Use the System

In the beginning, you will need to learn the remedy descriptions so that you know them thoroughly. Make a study of the books available (see page 75) to help you and further your understanding, always referring to Dr. Bach's "Twelve Healers & Other Remedies" if in any doubt. Once you KNOW the remedies you will know what information you need in order to make your selection. A clear knowledge of the remedies and an understanding of human nature, therefore, is all that is required to enable you to treat yourself with this system of healing and offer help to those you care for, who may also be in distress.

You will have noticed that some remedies describe the characteristics and personality of different people – for example Chicory, Agrimony, Vervain, Vine, Water Violet, Rock Water and Oak. We call remedies such as these "type remedies" because they are descriptive of types of people. Other remedies such as White Chestnut, Gentian, Aspen and Star of Bethlehem describe states of mind or moods which can be common to anyone, whatever their personality type may be. These are known as the "helper remedies" or "mood remedies".

One of the most common reactions when first confronted with the list of 38 remedies is to declare, "I need them all"! This is, however, quite a natural reaction and not at all unusual, because most of the remedy states, especially the mood remedies, are commonly experienced by us all at some time during our lives. They are the ups and downs of daily living and are therefore natural human emotions. Most of us are at some time or other troubled by something which makes us feel a little irritable, despondent, angry or frightened and we can usually "snap out of it" and think positively enough to restore the balance. On occasions, however, the mood seems to take hold and we are unable to shake it off. It gradually drags us down and we no longer feel happy or able to cope – we no longer feel ourselves. The appropriate remedies, taken just as the balance begins to waver, will help the mood to lift and thus restore inner harmony.

It is, however, often the case that a snowballing effect takes place, the roots of unhappiness begin to establish themselves and eventually what might have started off as a "bad mood" develops into a state of unbearable emotional anguish. It is then necessary to not only treat the anguish but to also look beneath it to discover the cause and how that particular person has responded to the disquiet in his or her life. This way, the emotional outlook can be placed into context to form a complete picture of the person as a whole. Each person will respond to different situations in a variety of ways, but those of a similar personality and character will react in a similar way. It is therefore the reaction to the event which provides a clue to the personality type and thus a guide to the appropriate "type remedy".

Recognising Type Remedies

During the course of your life you will have come across a mixture of people, all with different qualities which make them unique. Everybody is as vital and important as each other, like little cogs in the giant workings of life, and indeed, it would be a very boring world if we were all the same! The idiosyncrasies and characteristics of a particular person are what provides the overall impression of their nature, and each individual composition is depicted by one of the remedies. Whilst reading Chapter 2, some of the descriptions will have reminded you of people you know, or made you smile as you recognised yourself! We all know people who are extrovert and others who are introvert, those who are full of enthusiasm and those who are apathetic. We know immediately, therefore, by appreciating the basic personality, which group of remedies should be considered. Outspokenness for example would suggest remedies such as Vervain, Impatiens, Vine, Chicory, Oak, whereas those who are quiet would indicate "quieter" remedies such as Mimulus, Centaury, Larch or Water Violet. There are people who are very outgoing and talkative – they might be Agrimony if they are jolly and give the impression they haven't a care in the world, or Heather if their talkativeness is self-indulgent. As soon as we meet a person we are able to begin to form a picture of their make-up by the impression they give. For example, a great deal can be learned about a person's nature by the way they speak, the tone of their voice, what they choose to talk about, whether they are nervous, insistent or dreamy. Body language too can reveal a great deal. Impatiens types, for example, tend to talk quickly, may fidget and seem in a hurry, perhaps looking at their watch or interrupting with an answer before you have finished your question. If you have a discussion with someone who begins to get worked up about the particular topic, their eyes opening widely and their voice excited as they emphatically pursue their argument, then you may well be talking to a Vervain! Some people are instantly recognizable and are classic examples of a particular type remedy. Other people's personalities are more subtle, and sometimes you might find that there are those who seem to be a mixture of types. Equipped with a sound understanding of the remedies, however, you will know what questions you need to ask in order to extract the information you need to determine the correct choice.

As another example of the way different types of people respond to a given situation, let us consider seven students all about to take an examination together. Ann (Rock Rose) is absolutely terrified, sick with extreme nervousness and is literally shaking. Catherine (Agrimony) feels the same but pretends she doesn't. All her friends marvel at her apparent calmness and jovial attitude. David (Wild Rose) doesn't care whether he passes or fails. He hasn't bothered to study and has resigned himself to failure. Andrew (Impatiens) is biting his nails, watching the clock and tapping his foot in his eagerness and impatience to start his paper. Rosemary (Cerato) is so doubtful and uncertain about her interpretation of the subject that she seeks reassurance from the others, comparing their understanding with her own. Jennifer (Scleranthus) spends valuable time trying to decide which essay to write and so is still writing when time is up! Susan (Clematis), in the meantime, is gazing out of the window, daydreaming about the summer holidays, and doesn't notice that the examination has even commenced!

Set combination remedies for situations such as this are therefore inappropriate and although certain common remedies may often apply, every person is an individual and responds differently, so it is impossible to generalise. Even in illness people are affected in different ways. Some become very miserable and surrender to their ill-health. Others will soldier on regardless, despite their discomfort.

It is often helpful to test your understanding of the remedies by "prescribing" for people on television. Characters in a play often portray characteristics which illustrate their personality or display certain moods or emotions which can help you decide which remedy they may need. Or you can practise diagnosing type remedies for people in the public eye – politicians, TV personalities, sportsmen and women. Think about the members of your own family and your friends and consider their various traits, or if someone you know has been through a difficult period in the past, consider the effect this had, and relate their feelings to the remedies you would have given.

Using your understanding of the remedy descriptions,

see if you can recognize the remedy types involved in the following conversation:

ALAN: Would you like to come for a walk, Alison?

ALISON: Um… I don't know. Let me think about it.

ALAN: Well don't take all day! How about you Peter?

PETER: Yes, I'll come, but let me finish this first… and I've just got to telephone Fred about our meeting tomorrow – we're campaigning about the local residents' rights. It's so unfair how they're treated. Oh… and that reminds me, David should be drawing up a questionnaire… I must get on to him too… Give me five minutes and I'll be with you…

ALAN: Have you made up your mind yet Alison?

ALISON: I'm not sure whether I want to go or not. I can't decide.

ALAN: Well hurry up and make up your mind, we're nearly ready to go.

ALISON: Oh, you go. I'll stay here. No I won't – I'll come with you. Let me get my coat…

ALAN: Alright. Peter, are you ready?

PETER: Just about. Did I tell you about Jeff? The injustice that man has had to cope with – such a frustrating situation…

ALAN: Yes, yes, yes. Are you ready yet Alison?

ALISON: I've changed my mind. I don't think I will come after all.

ALAN: Let's go Peter.

PETER: Let me just ring David while it's fresh in
         my mind…

ALAN: Oh! I've wasted enough time, and I'd prefer to
         go by myself anyway. Goodbye you two!

Alison clearly needs Scleranthus – she's full of indecision
and cannot make up her mind. Alan (Impatiens) is very
impatient and has no time for Alison's hesitancy. Peter is so
engrossed in his attempts to put the world to rights, that
although he would have gone for a walk with Alan, he was
not able to give it his full attention. His principles and
earnest enthusiasm indicate his Vervain nature.

Dr. Bach described some of the remedies by way of a
story, each character representing a different remedy and
illustrating the positive side of the nature as well as the
characteristic negative outlook. He called it "The Story of
the Travellers":

> *"Once upon a time; and it is always once upon a time,
> sixteen travellers set out to journey through a forest.*
>
> *At first all went well, but after they had journeyed some
> distance, one of the number, Agrimony, began to be
> worried as to whether they were on the right path. Later in
> the afternoon as they went deeper into the shadows,
> Mimulus began to be afraid, afraid that they had lost the
> road. When the sun set and the shadows deepened and the
> night noises of the forest were heard around them, Rock
> Rose became full of terror and was in a state of panic. In
> the middle of the night when all was blackness, Gorse lost
> all hope and said, 'I can go no further; you go along, but I
> shall stay here as I am until death relieves my sufferings.'*
>
> *Oak, on the other hand, though feeling all was lost and
> that they would never again see the sunshine said, 'I shall*

struggle on to the very last', and he did in a wild way.

Scleranthus had some hope but at times he suffered so from uncertainty and indecision, first wanting to take one road and almost at once another. Clematis plodded on quietly and patiently, but caring oh so little if he fell into the last sound sleep or whether he got out of the forest. Gentian at times much cheered the party, but at others fell into a state of despondency and depression.

Others of the travellers never feared but that they would get through and in their own way wanted so much to help their companions.

Heather was very sure he knew the path and wanted all the company to take his way. Chicory had no concern about the end of the journey but was full of solicitude as to whether his fellows were footsore or tired or had enough to eat. Cerato had not much confidence in his judgement and wanted to try every path to be sure they were not wrong, and meek little Centaury so wanted to lighten the burden that he was ready to carry everybody's baggage. Unfortunately for little Centaury, he generally carried the burden of those most able to bear their own because they called the loudest.

Rock Water, all afire to help, a little depressed the party because he would criticise what they were doing wrong, and yet Rock Water knew the way. Vervain should also have known the path well enough, but although he had become a little confused, held forth at length as to the only way out of the wood. Impatiens, too, well knew the pathway home, so well that he was impatient with those less speedy than himself. Water Violet had travelled that way before and knew the right road and yet was a little proud and a little disdainful that others did not *understand. Water Violet thought them a little inferior.*

And in the end they all came through the forest.

Now they go as guides to other travellers who have not made the journey before, and, because they know there is a pathway through, and because they know the darkness of the forest is but the shadows of the night, they walk as 'gentlemen unafraid', and each of the sixteen sojourners teach in their own way the lesson, the example needed.

Agrimony strides along free of all care, and jests on everything. Mimulus can know no fear; Rock Rose in the darkest moments is just a picture of calm, serene courage. Gorse in the blackest night tells them of the progress they will make when the sun rises in the morning.

Oak stands steadfast in the strongest gale; Scleranthus walks with perfect certainty; the eyes of Clematis are fixed with joy on the journey's end, and no difficulties or setbacks can discourage Gentian.

Heather has learnt that each traveller must walk in his own way and quietly strides in front to show it can be done. Chicory, always waiting to lend a hand, but only when asked, and then so quietly. Cerato knows so well the little paths that lead to nowhere, and Centaury ever seeks the weakest who find their burden heavy.

Rock Water has forgotten to accuse, he just spends all the time encouraging. Vervain no longer preaches but silently points the way. Impatiens knows no hurry but lingers amongst the hindmost to keep their pace; and Water Violet, more like an angel than a man, passes amongst the company like a breath of warm wind or a ray of glorious sunshine, blessing everyone."

Edward Bach 1934

CHOOSING REMEDIES FOR OTHERS

"Amongst the remedies, you will find those which will apply to all the conditions that can be met. Such as some for those who suffer from uncertainty, never knowing quite what they wish or what is right for them. Some for loneliness; others for those who are too sensitive. Others for depression and so on.

And with very little effort it becomes easy to find the remedy or remedies which a patient needs to help them."

Edward Bach 1936

As suggested earlier in this chapter, try to relate your understanding of the remedies to those whom you know and to experiences you have encountered. This will help to consolidate what you have learned and give you confidence in your ability to prescribe.

The first remedy you are most likely to use is Rescue Remedy because emergency situations are generally those which call for prompt action and as the Rescue Remedy is specifically prepared for this purpose, there is no need to consider reasons, reactions or moods – Dr. Bach did this for us when he provided the Rescue Remedy composite.

Rescue Remedy, however, is not a panacea and so other remedies should be considered when a more specific emotional outlook is apparent. For example, if you are filled with dismay after some disappointing news, the remedy to give you encouragement and restore your faith is Gentian. Rescue Remedy would not be appropriate in this case. For clear descending moods such as this, it is not difficult to select the required remedy, and if a friend or relative should need some help to regain their happiness or peace of mind, the right remedy will not be hard to find.

When a problem is more deep-rooted, however, further consideration is necessary because it is on these occasions that many of the remedy states seem to be indicated and some discussion is required in order to "peel the onion" and thereby discover the underlying problem.

Quite often it soon becomes obvious when the difficulty first began. People frequently say, "I have suffered this way since I retired", or "We were burgled a few years ago and ever since then I have suffered with panic attacks", or "When we moved house I was unable to settle and have now lost all my confidence". If you can establish a definite cause for the present difficulties, the appropriate remedy should be included even if the incident occurred many years ago because the effect has clearly lingered. For true healing to take place this must be treated. Shock for example can be so delayed that several weeks, months or even years might pass before any sign becomes apparent. In the meantime, however, the shock trapped or locked away inside begins to fester, and although help may be eventually sought to relieve the subsequent manifestation of depression, guilt or fear, unless the original shock is treated and eradicated, healing cannot be complete. Remedies to help the depression, guilt or fear (or whatever it might be) will also be necessary, just as attention to a stomach ulcer would be necessary to relieve the immediate pain and suffering, but it is not sufficient to only treat the resulting mood, just as it is insufficient to only treat the ulcer. The cause is always the most important factor.

It is not always clear, however, what the true cause of the problem is. For some, the present state of mind is one which has its roots in childhood or one which has developed over such a long period that they have lost sight of its origin. In these cases, simply treat the state of mind or mood which is apparent NOW. As time progresses and the remedies begin to work, the outer layers of the onion will gradually be shed and the underlying emotions will begin to surface until eventually the root cause is revealed and can be treated.

Let us consider an example. Suppose someone came to you for help complaining of anxiety. "Anxiety" itself is not enough on which to base your Bach Remedy prescription. You will therefore need to ask in what way they are anxious, what are they anxious about, and how it affects them as well as ascertaining what might have caused it in the first place. They might reply that they are anxious about their work, their children or their health, and it will depend upon their answers as to which remedy or remedies are required. Let us suppose that this person is anxious about their health. This would immediately suggest that there is a fear of illness and if this proves to be the case, Mimulus is the remedy required (it is a known fear). But during the course of discussion, it may become apparent that this person cannot bear the thought of illness because it makes him or her feel unclean or diseased. Further investigation may reveal that this person is obsessive about cleanliness in the home, always making sure the cushions are placed correctly and the pictures absolutely straight. This state of mind and personality type would indicate Crab Apple. Both remedies would therefore be necessary to correct the imbalance and thus help to free this person from their anxiety.

Let us now take this one step further and again consider our anxious patient. This time let us suppose his or her state of mind has created some physical suffering and the person in this case seeks help for eczema, complaining that the skin eruption coincided with the mounting anxiety. It is the anxiety that we are interested in, not the eczema – it is the person we treat not the disease – and so the same process of uncovering the reasons for the anxiety and so on are necessary. Another person suffering with eczema might require entirely different remedies so each case must be considered on its own merits and each person treated as an individual.

Consultations

The most important consideration when conducting an interview is to encourage the person you are helping to do the talking. And as they talk, make a note of the remedies which come to mind. The odd pertinent question here and there to clarify a point or steer the conversation towards an area which is important to the treatment is all that should be necessary.

Quite often people will, understandably, feel a little nervous, especially if they do not know you, so it is important to always make them feel at ease. After an initial introduction you might like to ask whether they know very much about Dr. Bach's work. If not, you can briefly explain the principles of the therapy to help them understand how it works and therefore what to expect.

If the person you are treating has difficulty expressing their emotional outlook in terms of their difficulty or illness, it will be necessary to approach the matter in a more subtle, indirect way, perhaps asking about their family, work, holidays, neighbours and so on. General conversation such as this will offer the opportunity for you to pursue areas of disquiet and this may then lead to the true essence of the problem. If people wish to talk about their physical complaints, and immediately launch into a lengthy account of their ailments allow them to do so. It can be helpful from their point of view because they are given an opportunity to explain their pain or discomfort, and for the practitioner, it can provide a lot of helpful information because you are able to study the way in which they explain their difficulties. If necessary, you can interject with a question such as "Does it get you down?", and this will then guide the conversation in an emotional direction. Or ask when the problem began and what may have been going on in the person's life around that time. This too will offer an opportunity to discuss emotional feelings.

Once you have reached a decision regarding your choice of remedies, you may go through them with the person you are treating. Occasionally it might be more appropriate to prepare the medicine without discussing its contents, but generally I feel it is important to explain which remedies are given because the person can then understand WHY he or she is taking them. The recognition of the problem and the desire to put it right is the first step towards that inner healing and if the selection is unknown, an important aspect of this healing process is lost. If however the person can return home comforted by having shared their problems, and with a remedy that they understand and which provides some practical help, then there will be hope. That in itself will lift the spirits and then the first stage of healing will have occurred.

CHOOSING REMEDIES FOR ONESELF

Although the remedies are straightforward and simple to understand, many people find it more difficult to treat themselves than to treat others. This is not so unusual because it can be hard, especially when spirits are low, to be objective about oneself and think clearly enough to recognize the remedies which are required. Perhaps we know ourselves too well (or not well enough!) and find that nearly all the remedy states seem to apply. This is why many people prefer to seek the help of a friend or practitioner to guide them. However, the remedies are intended primarily as a means of self-help and therefore self-diagnosis should not present a problem.

If you do experience difficulty, I suggest that you first of all make a note of the remedies you feel you need, and then ask yourself the same questions that you would ask someone else if you were helping them. Why are you afraid? In what way are you anxious? What do you worry about? "Why" is such an important word because it is the answer to "why?" that will lead you to the required remedy or remedies. For example you may feel you are lacking in self-confidence (Larch) but the reason why may be due to fear and lack of courage (Mimulus). By going through your choice of remedies in this way and considering the reasons for choosing each one, you will be able to eliminate the unnecessary remedies from your initial list. Remember – treat the cause and not the effect! Quite often the "effect" is manifested by superficial emotions which tend to clutter the true picture. These will begin to fade once treatment of the cause has commenced.

It is also important of course to consider your personality as a whole so that your remedy choice can be based on a complete picture. You will know whether you are timid or outgoing; strong-willed or give in easily; sociable or reserved and so on. Think about yourself – the way you respond to criticism; how you might feel if you were cheated; how you feel at parties, meetings or other social occasions; how you react when you are driving, and how you deal with illness or pain. Your actions, feelings and responses to these situations, and whether or not you show the way you feel, are all important clues in helping you determine your particular type remedy. You should then consider your mood or emotional upset in relation to and in context with your general outlook and personality. This too will help you to eliminate unnecessary remedies by forming a clearer picture of your difficulties. You do, of course, have to be completely honest with yourself and be able to admit when you feel resentful or jealous, intolerant or suspicious. There are some descriptions which may sound "nicer" than others, but all the remedies describe natural human emotions, common to us all, so don't be ashamed of your feelings. The fact that you have recognized them is the first step towards your own inner healing, and the appropriate remedy is there to help you.

You might find it helpful to write your feelings down as though you were writing to a hypothetical practitioner. Sometimes this in itself helps to focus your mind on the basis of the problem, but in any case, the written word can then be studied more objectively and the remedies chosen accordingly. Many people find this a helpful exercise as they find written expression flows more easily, and it can often prove therapeutic in itself, especially if the problem is something which has been suppressed over a period of time. Writing it down becomes a release and often acts as a platform from which you can look at yourself and your emotional outlook in a more detached way.

Another method of selecting the appropriate remedies for yourself is to consider what virtue you feel is lacking, and therefore which quality you most wish to develop or correct. For example you may wish you could be more certain of what you want to do in life. Consider this and again ask yourself why you feel uncertain. Wild Oat, Scleranthus or Cerato may apply so read up on each one and select that which most aptly describes you. Or you might feel that you would like to be more understanding of others' misfortune (Beech) or that you would like to be a better listener (Heather) and so on. You may be able to ask a close friend how he or she sees you – again a degree of honesty is needed! Do they think you are too hesitant, too impatient, too nervous, are you bossy or easily manipulated? To balance the negative characteristics, you can also ask which positive qualities he or she sees you possess – are you patient, or brave, do you make friends easily, are you a strong leader or are you gentle, kind and willing to serve? As Nora Weeks would say, "Ask for a true opinion of yourself and do not mind what you are told"!

It is true that treatment with the Bach Remedies involves a rather different approach to that of any other therapy. Medicine, generally, treats symptoms and diseases and even truly holistic medicine such as homoeopathy, takes into account the physical aspects as well. The Bach Remedies, however, concentrate entirely on the personality and emotions and sometimes people find it difficult to reconcile this approach with their malady. But as Dr. Bach explained in "The Twelve Healers and Other Remedies",

> *"The mind being the most delicate and sensitive part of the body, shows the onset and the course of disease much more definitely than the body, so that the outlook of mind is chosen as the guide as to which remedy or remedies are necessary."*

CHOOSING REMEDIES FOR CHILDREN

Sometimes people wonder how the remedies can be applied to children, especially young children and babies, because they cannot always express their feelings. However, it is again a matter of treating the person and so the nature of the child should be considered as a whole. The mood of the child is often apparent, displayed through their behaviour. Consider how the child acts when playing – does he/she become annoyed when a jigsaw piece does not fit, or the building bricks will not balance? Does he or she knock them all down in a temper or quickly lose interest? Is the child patient, caring or oversensitive? Is he or she independent or possessive? Boisterous or subdued? All these indicators help us to find the correct remedies. For example, a very active child who is always doing something, never sitting still, would require Impatiens, and perhaps Vervain. A child who is gentle and considerate and always does as he or she is told, and is easily bossed by other children would require Centaury, and/or Mimulus if very shy, timid or fearful. Vine would help the child who is bossy or bullying and is very demanding and strong. A very sleepy child may be of the Clematis nature; sulkiness would indicate Willow; Chicory if constantly demanding attention.

When a child is ill, the mood can be observed and the remedies chosen accordingly. The way they behave when unwell is often the key to their temperament and one of the best indicators of their type remedy. It was this observation which led Dr. Bach to the conclusion that the mind, the emotions and therefore the person should be treated, not only the disease.

He said:

> *"If Tommy gets measles, he might be irritable, Sissy may be quiet and drowsy, Johnny wants to be petted, little Peter may be all nerves and fearful, Bobby wants to be left alone and so on. If the disease has such different effects it is certain it is no use treating the disease alone. It is better to treat Tommy, Sissy, Johnny, Peter and Bobby and get them each well – and goodbye the measles!"*

For babies, again one needs to consider the behaviour and temperament – a contented, happy, laughing baby would need Agrimony when restless. Babies who cry and want to be cuddled are difficult to put to bed at night because they do not want to be left alone, and always demanding Mum's attention would need Chicory. Impatiens if they become irritated and impatient, and so on.

Rescue Remedy is generally calming and is therefore helpful on many occasions, particularly when shock, terror or extreme fretfulness is apparent. But do seek the advice of your Health Visitor or doctor if the problem persists.

During childhood, a great deal of growth and developmental changes take place during a short period of time. Walnut is therefore often a helpful remedy during the various milestones of a child's development – teething, walking, talking, going to school and puberty for example. The notorious temper tantrums at two or three years are often created by frustration – the child's mental development outstripping their physical capabilities.

Always the child's individual temperament and personality must be taken into account, but generally speaking, for these outbursts, Holly is a helpful remedy for temper and spite, Walnut for the growth changes, Beech for intolerance, Impatiens for the irritation and impatience, and Vervain for tension and frustration.

There are many other situations when the remedies can be of help. Going to school for the first time or starting a new school can often be a traumatic experience. Rescue Remedy is helpful on such occasions, along with Walnut for adjustment, together with others which might apply depending on the individual child's specific needs, such as Larch if there is a lack of self-confidence. For nightmares,

Rock Rose is needed (or Rescue Remedy as this contains Rock Rose), and Honeysuckle if it is due to a recurrent upsetting memory. Another difficult period is often when a new brother or sister arrives. Some children adjust very well and accept the new baby without any problem, but others become jealous or feel threatened or unloved when they realise that the little bundle which is always in Mum's arms is there to stay! Holly would be the remedy to help the jealousy, Chicory if they feel ignored, and Willow for resentment and sulkiness.

The next major milestone is adolescence when a lot of growth changes again take place. As well as Walnut for adjustment, Crab Apple is often helpful because there is frequently a degree of embarrassment surrounding the changing appearance. Crab Apple can also be applied externally if the child is troubled with a blemished skin (dilute 2 drops in an egg cup of water and dab on after washing). This period of development can often give rise to many negative moods as the child becomes an adult. During their search for independence; their own needs and desires, emotions can become quite stormy! Appropriate remedies for the states of mind which become apparent will help in these turbulent years.

As we grow up, we accumulate experience, and these experiences fuse with our basic nature to form our adult attitudes and character. As we grow older we become more aware of the various hurdles of life, and each one we tackle teaches us something about ourselves. These trials and tribulations can interfere with or block our healing processes and so when we take remedies to help us, sometimes we find a barrier has developed making the remedies' job that little bit harder. With children, however, there is no barrier and so their recovery is generally that much quicker. We have, I'm sure, all seen children playing happily and running about, their faces still spotty from measles or chicken pox! Children therefore respond very well to the remedies and they do not usually need many doses to become "themselves" again.

CHOOSING REMEDIES FOR ANIMALS AND PLANTS

Animals

As with children, animals usually respond extremely well to the remedies. To prescribe, once again, the temperament of the animal concerned needs to be considered together with its particular mood and nature generally. A dog, for example, may bark viciously at passers-by, but the reasons for the barking may vary a great deal. Some may bark because they are afraid (Mimulus or Rock Rose), others because they are possessive (Chicory) and are guarding their master, others because they are ruling their territory and are displaying their dominance (Vine). Others may seem to bark or snarl purely out of malice and one may think in terms of Holly for this, but it is the underlying cause which is the most important issue and the real guide. The dog may of course be the victim of another dog's aggression and so remedies such as Centaury and Mimulus would be applicable.

When an animal is ill, its mood will often change. Mournful eyes which look at you as if to say, "Feel sorry for me, I'm not well" belong to an animal who needs Willow; drowsiness and apathy call for Clematis and Wild Rose; irritability may indicate Impatiens, and aggression often indicates Vine.

All animals are like humans, animals are individuals and

need to be considered as such, even though certain species or breeds might share similar tendencies. For example, many cats may be Water Violet types (proud and independent), but each one would have a temperament peculiar to itself.

Rescue Remedy is always useful to include when treating animals because so often shock or terror is a major cause of their troubles. The dosage is as for humans – 4 drops of Rescue Remedy/2 drops of other remedies. The remedy can be diluted into a little water or into a treatment bottle so that doses can be administered throughout the day or may simply be added to the animal's drinking bowl, food, or on a biscuit. For larger animals such as horses, 10 drops are recommended, added to a bucket of water, or the usual 4 drops on a cube of sugar. Try to administer the drops as often as you can, but at least 4 times daily.

Plants

The health and well-being of plant-life is generally confined to the auspices of gardening manuals, and the idea of treating a plant medicinally, and in particular emotionally, may appear to be a little strange – perhaps even eccentric. But plants, like all living things, are part of Nature and so they too have an inner Life Force which responds to the healing energies that Nature yields.

Although plants are usually the providers of medicines for the ills of mankind, Nature works both ways. They who give shall also receive! Anyone who has kept plants in the garden or in the house will have seen some sad drooping leaves, or noticed a plant struggling against disease. More commonly (unless you are a very lucky gardener!), you will have had experience of plants that have not responded well to re-potting or re-locating, and seem to have difficulty adjusting to change of soil or environment, or suffering a certain amount of shock which weakens their natural ability to survive after transplantation. The Bach Remedies can therefore be of great benefit to plants, and there have been many reported successes.

Prescribing for plants, however, may seem at first a little difficult, if not unusual. After all, one cannot ask them questions or expect them to express their feelings as we would do. Nevertheless, they do display their outlook through their appearance, and it is on this expression of need that you should base your choice of remedies. A plant that looks very droopy and sorry for itself, for example, would need Willow; one which has given up on life and appears to be dying may be revived with Gorse, and Crab Apple if there is sign of disease. For re-potting, transplanting and for cuttings try Walnut (for the adjustment) and Star of Bethlehem (for shock), as well as individual remedies which you may feel apply. Plants which have been in a dark position and have struggled to reach the light would require Olive to replenish their lost energy resources. And of course Rescue Remedy, to alleviate trauma, shock and fright, is always recommended.

To administer remedies to plants, simply add 10 drops to a watering can (it does not matter if other plants are watered too – the remedies can only help!), or the usual 2 drops (4 of Rescue Remedy) to the individual plant's water. It is, of course, important not to OVER-water because to do so would create further complications, but this may be difficult to avoid if the plant requires frequent remedy doses. However, the problem can be overcome by administering the drops daily in a dessert-spoon of water. This way the plant will gain the benefit of regular remedies without becoming too wet. In addition, the leaves may be sprayed with a dilution of remedies, and this may be especially useful if the leaves appear unhealthy or dry. A combination of Rescue Remedy and Crab Apple would be ideal when used in this way.

CHAPTER FOUR

REMEDY PREPARATION AND ADMINISTRATION

How The Remedies Are Made

The Bach Remedies are prepared quite simply – no complicated technique is involved or vast equipment required. The method is explained in detail in "The Bach Remedies, Illustrations and Preparation" by Nora Weeks and Victor Bullen, but I will briefly describe it here.

There are two methods: the first through the action of the sun and the second by boiling. The sun method is unique to Dr. Bach and involves placing the flowering heads of the plants concerned on the surface of a small glass bowl filled with pure spring water. The bowl is then left in the sunshine for three hours during which time the water becomes impregnated with the healing properties of the plant. The flower heads, having transferred their vital energy to the water, are then discarded. The water which holds the life force of the plant is preserved in brandy (Dr. Bach's own chosen preservative), and becomes known as the Mother Tincture.

Dr. Bach developed this method during the early part of his discovery. In the beginning he prepared his remedies homoeopathically but wanted to evolve a method which could be easily understood by all so that those who wished to try could prepare a remedy for themselves. One morning, he noticed the dew which had formed on the flower petals, glistening in the early morning sunshine, and wondered whether the healing vibrations of the flower had been drawn out into the dewdrop by the warmth of the sun. When he found that it had, the next day he set about collecting all the dew, tapping it into bottles, and this is how some of his first remedies were prepared. But he soon realised that collecting dew was not very practical and of course extremely time consuming! Eventually, after a lot of thought, he decided to try creating his own, much larger "dewdrop", filling a thin glass bowl with water from a nearby spring. This marked the birth of Dr. Bach's unique sun method of preparation and is how 20 of the flower remedies have been prepared ever since.

The other 18 are made by boiling, and those prepared by this method are mostly (although not all) the trees. Short lengths of twigs filled with the flower or catkins are collected and boiled in pure spring water for half an hour and then left to cool. Again the twigs with their leaves and flowers are discarded having transferred their healing properties to the water during the boiling process. This method is more akin to a homoeopathic preparation but Dr. Bach found this to be the most appropriate means of extracting the vitality from these particular 18 remedies.

The next stage in the preparation of the remedies is to dilute the Mother Tincture into a further quantity of brandy. This liquid is then known as the "stock" remedy, and although it is a dilution of the original tincture, it is nevertheless considered to be a concentrated remedy because it requires further dilution before administration.

The Dr. Bach Centre, Mount Vernon, has been the nucleus of the work since Dr. Bach came to live there in 1934. His remedies have always been made at the Centre according to Dr. Bach's instructions and with much loving care by the trustees and curators of his work. The Bach Centre is a small and humble cottage situated in the heart of a picturesque village in the Oxfordshire countryside. The history of the growth of Dr. Bach's work can be found in "The Story of Mount Vernon" which describes how Nora Weeks and Victor Bullen steadfastly fulfilled their promise to continue the Doctor's work as was his express wish. When Dr. Bach settled at Mount Vernon, he had already discovered half the series of 38 remedies and it was during these final two and a half years of his life that he found the last 19, all growing within a small radius of Mount Vernon. To his delight he found his first 19 remedies (with two exceptions – Olive and Vine) growing locally too, and many of these actual locations are still used today in the preparation of the Bach Flower Remedies.

MAKING UP A TREATMENT

All the Bach Remedies are available individually as "stock" remedies. This means they are a concentrated remedy preserved in brandy, and will therefore keep indefinitely. It is from the stock remedy that the medicine or treatment is prepared.

The method of preparation of a treatment is largely one of preference. The Bach Remedies are harmless and so one cannot overdose. If too much remedy is taken it will do no harm. Similarly, if the wrong or inappropriate remedy is taken it will not cause any ill-effects. Having understood how the mother tinctures are prepared, you will realise that no physical part of the plant is ingested and as all Dr. Bach's remedy plants are non-poisonous, they do not contain any substance which would be capable of producing any adverse reaction. There is, however, one point which should be mentioned here and that is the brandy content. As you will see from the following paragraphs, only a very small amount of the stock remedy is taken as a treatment, but even so, there are some people who may be very sensitive to even this minute quantity, or those who cannot take alcohol for religious reasons. It is important, therefore, to bear this in mind when treating others with the remedies.

There are basically two methods of making up a treatment. The drops may either be diluted into a glass of water and sipped at intervals which would be the most appropriate method if you are dealing with emergencies or passing moods, or made up as a treatment bottle which would be more suitable if the problem is long-term or deep-rooted.

To make up a treatment bottle, you will need an empty 30ml bottle with a dropper. If a 30ml size cannot be obtained, a slightly smaller bottle will suffice. Most large chemists stock empty dropper bottles. You will also need some mineral or (still) spring water which is available in bottles from most health food stores or supermarkets. Make sure the bottle is clean and free from any contaminants, and then having selected the required remedies, simply add two drops from each one to the empty bottle. Fill this up with the spring/mineral water and screw on the dropper cap. This bottle represents your treatment, and from it you take 4 drops at least 4 times daily. This is the minimum requirement, but if necessary, such as when the mood is acute, the drops can be taken more frequently. Mineral or spring water should be chosen when making up a treatment bottle because the preparation has the potential of lasting some two or three weeks. Bottled waters will stay fresh for quite some time and will therefore last for the duration of the treatment. Tap water, unfortunately, will usually deteriorate and go stale very quickly. However, if you have no access to bottled water, then it is quite alright to use tap water, preferably filtered, but add a teaspoon of brandy or other spirit to the preparation to help preserve the water content. A little brandy should also be added to a treatment containing even bottled water if it is likely to be stored in a warm place or climate. If you can, try to store your diluted remedy in the fridge.

The drops can be taken directly onto the tongue from the pipette, or in a little water if preferred. They can even be added to a cup of tea or other beverage if more convenient. If you can, try to hold the dose in the mouth for a second or two before swallowing and try to visualise the positive energy you are taking, like a breath of fresh air.

Try to limit the choice of remedies to about six. This is not because the remedies would counteract each other or cause some ill-effect, but simply because too many remedies taken together tend to cloud the issue and are unable to work quite so well. However, again everyone is an individual and needs vary from person to person. Sometimes only one or two remedies are needed in which case only those chosen should be given. But on other occasions seven or eight may be indicated, and if all these are required, then it is better to take them all than to exclude an essential remedy, because to do so would mean that an important element of the complete healing may be missed. As time progresses, however, and improvement takes place, some remedies can be omitted from the subsequent treatment if they have done their work and are no longer required. Similarly if other moods become prevalent during the course of treatment, the appropriate remedy should be added. This is often the case because as the healing process begins, a certain cleansing takes place, and emotions which may have lain dormant for a long time, having been suppressed and therefore not really experienced, begin to surface. Just as the water of a muddy pool can appear to be clean and clear, in order to get rid of the silt which has settled on the bottom we have to disturb the water and it will become cloudy for a little while until all the debris rises to the surface and can be scooped away.

Some people find it more convenient to simply take the drops from the stock remedy in a glass of water, and this would be the more suitable method in an emergency or when the mood is short lived and does not represent a culmination of emotions. Instead of making up a treatment bottle, simply take 2 drops of each required remedy in a glass of water (the size does not matter). This should then be sipped at intervals until the mood has lifted. Longer term treatment can be taken this way too of course, and each glass of remedy can be allowed to last all day, taking a sip from it every couple of hours. This method is a little less economical because the glass will need to be replenished every day or after a few hours, whereas a treatment bottle would last a couple of weeks, or at least a few days. However, because no overdose is possible with the Bach Remedies, the choice of treatment preparation is entirely one of personal preference.

Whichever method you choose, take your first dose when you get up in the morning, and your last dose before retiring to bed in the evening. You may also wish to keep it by the bedside if you are prone to waking in the night.

For babies, diluted dosage drops can be added to a bottle of juice or feed, or given on a teaspoon. If the baby is being breastfed only, the mother, by taking remedies herself, will pass their effects on to her baby through her milk. But of course breast milk takes a little time to develop, so if the need is immediate it would be more appropriate to give the diluted drops directly by spoon.

As we have seen previously, Rescue Remedy is a ready-prepared composite in stock remedy form and because of this, the dosage is 4 drops instead of 2 as with the other remedies. The method of treatment preparation is otherwise exactly the same, and it can be added to a treatment mixture if necessary, but because Rescue Remedy is intended for emergencies, the most appropriate method would be to take it in a glass or cup of water, sipped slowly until relief is obtained or the shock or panic subsides. If, for some reason, liquid is not available – perhaps whilst out shopping or taking a walk – then the remedy can be taken neat, straight from the stock bottle – 4 drops just the same. However, don't forget that the stock remedies are preserved in brandy so it will taste quite strong! Rescue Remedy can also be applied to the lips, temples, wrists and behind the ears if it cannot be taken orally, and relief will still be obtained.

Rescue Remedy, and other appropriate remedies if necessary, can be helpful for external traumas too. A few drops of Rescue Remedy applied to the skin after a minor burn will relieve the pain straight away. Alternatively, a dilution in lukewarm or tepid water can be used as a lotion to bathe the affected area. Rescue Remedy cream is also very soothing and healing and can be used externally for a variety of occasions, from a nettle sting to general massage.

How the Remedies Work

Having understood the way the remedies are made, we know that no physical part of the plant remains once preparation is complete and therefore no physical part of the plant is ingested. It is therefore sometimes a little difficult to comprehend exactly how the remedies actually work and it is a question which has often been asked.

First of all it is important to appreciate energy as a life

force of which all of Nature is a part and to which we all belong. The healing property within a flower may therefore be considered to be the outlet of the Life Force of that plant; in effect the soul or spirit of the plant. And because it is an intrinsic thing, just as our spirit or soul is to us, it cannot be handled, injured or destroyed.

Everything in life has a purpose, from the simplest forms to the most complex, each one having a part to play in the workings of the great machinery of life. Plants contribute in a variety of ways. Some provide food, others act as a host to parasitic life forms, others nourish the soil or provide oxygen. Others have the ability to heal. Most herbal preparations procure the medicinal properties by extracting the oil or by drying the leaves or the root. Dr. Bach's remedies are an extract of the healing life of the plant which is non-physical and therefore something abstract. It cannot be measured or analysed like a chemical or drug, and so the potent element cannot be extracted and identified. To attempt to examine the healing properties in a scientific way would be like adopting a scientific approach to explain why we are moved by certain music or why we might feel peaceful by the sea. These phenomena cannot be broken down for analysis, yet they do nevertheless exist. It is the same with the remedies. Their healing energies simply lift our vibrations and unblock the channels within our minds so that we can approach life more positively. And with the return of inner strength and harmony, the body's own natural healing processes are able to begin.

The remedies therefore help us to help ourselves. So think of them not as a medicine but as part of life – part of you. Take them as you need them, just as you would eat when you are hungry or drink when you are thirsty. If you feel afraid, take Mimulus, if you feel impatient take Impatiens. It is as simple as that!

THE HEALING PERIOD

People often ask for how long they should take the remedies and how soon they should expect to see some improvement. There is no single definite answer because each person is a separate entity and every situation unique. Each one of us will have a slightly different approach and so there are many considerations to take into account. Generally, however, passing moods and emotions which have developed suddenly or recently will not take long to correct. Perhaps only a few doses will be required. But for problems which have become deep-rooted and firmly established, perhaps evolving over a period of several months, years or even decades, healing will be a much more gradual process and will naturally take longer.

Often it is in hindsight that one notices an improvement has taken place. And because the remedies act in such a subtle and gentle way, sometimes a change in mood occurs without our noticing. Our true self begins to emerge once more, and like meeting an old friend, the familiarity and comforting inner glow soon returns. This is, of course, as it should be, and so it does not feel at all unusual. After all, it is the negativity – the depression, anxiety, anger – which seems unnatural. The positive aspect which we strive to achieve – the confidence, courage, even-temper, joy – is already naturally within us. So when it is re-awakened, we do not become different people, just ourselves again.

The answer, therefore, is already within us, but we can help our own healing process with positive thought. And although this might be difficult in the beginning, the remedies will help us to feel more optimistic and thus give us hope and lift our spirits. Ill-health is rather like a flight of stairs. The longer and more severe the suffering, the longer and steeper the staircase. But as we take the remedies, we begin to climb, one step at a time, until eventually we reach the top. We might take each step slowly or we might leap up the first few quickly and easily. We might stop every so often to catch our breath. Each one of us will approach the staircase in a different way, but however we tackle it, progress is always forward. There are remedies to help us if we lose our way, or find ourselves turning back, or if we are uncertain and feel afraid about taking the next step.

Life is full of challenges – pleasant as well as unpleasant – but whatever it is that presents a stumbling block in our lives, it is there for a purpose, to help us learn about life and give us experience. There is something for us to understand from all experiences, good and bad, and always something to gain, for no matter how negative a situation might seem, there is always a positive aspect to consider. Having endured the suffering, whatever it might be, it is then up to us to take heed of these warning signs should they ever return, and correct the imbalance before it has a chance to make us feel so unwell again. And that is our lesson. The remedies are there to help and guide us, but true progress – our real healing – comes from within.

CHAPTER FIVE

FURTHER READING

This book will have provided a good basic understanding of the principles and practice methods of the Bach system of healing. The keyword is "simpolicity" and the subject is not complex so a vast amount of reading is not necessary. However, there is much more to learn about the Bach Remedies than can be provided here, so here is a list of other books which will help further your understanding of Dr. Bach and his work:

The Essential Writings of Dr Edward Bach
by Dr Edward Bach with a preface by Judy Ramsell Howard
This book brings together two short works written by Dr Bach himself. *The Twelve Healers* explains simply and clearly each of the flower remedy states. The title can sometimes be a little confusing, but it originated when Dr Bach's discovery was only in its infancy and there were only 12 remedies. The title was retained because it had become familiar to readers, but it does nevertheless include descriptions of all 38 remedies.

Heal Thyself outlines Dr Bach's philosophy, and although not about the remedies themselves, it helps one's understanding of how they work, and describes his belief of the true cause of disease.

Illustrated Handbook of the Bach Flower Remedies
by Philip M. Chancellor

This book, although compiled by Philip Chancellor, contains Nora Weeks's descriptions of each remedy as originally published in the Bach Remedy Newsletters. Each remedy description is supplemented by several of her case histories which help the learner appreciate their use. It is a comprehensive book and an extremely helpful aid to understanding the remedies in more depth.

Dictionary of the Bach Flower Remedies
by T. W. Hyne Jones

This is, in effect, an abridged version of the Handbook, giving key sentences to describe the positive and negative aspects of each remedy. It is helpful as a quick reference guide.

Bach Flower Remedies for Women by Judy Ramsell Howard

An open account of womanhood and the trials encountered by women of all ages covering subjects such as menstruation, pregnancy, fertility, dieting, screening, menopause etc., and providing constructive advice on how the Bach Flower remedies can fit into a woman's life and help to relieve the associated emotional traumas.

The Bach Remedies Workbook by Stefan Ball

Here is a self-contained course in the selection and use of the Bach Flower Remedies. It starts from first principles and in seven progressive sections covers all 38 of the Bach Flower Remedies and the states of mind and emotions that they can be used to help.

Practical exercises, quizzes, games and suggestions for further work help readers gain a comprehensive grasp of Dr. Bach's famous system.

Bach Flower Remedies for Animals by Stefan Ball &
Judy Ramsell Howard
The Bach Flower Remedies offer every owner the opportunity to take care of the psychological health of his or her pet. An animal that is feeling well in itself is a healthy animal which will recover quickly from illness.

Instant help is at hand your animal with an acute psychological disorder, change in behaviour, emergencies of all kinds and support in difficult situations. Precise information is given on preparation, dosage and dispensing.

All of the above titles are published by Vermilion. The following are availabe from The Dr. Edward Bach Centre, Mount Vernon, Sotwell, Wallingford, Oxon. OX10 0PZ, United Kingdom:

The Story of Mount Vernon by Judy Ramsell Howard
This provides an account of the continuation of Dr. Bach's work since his death in 1936, and is therefore a form of sequel to the Medical Discoveries. Dr. Bach's devoted helpers Nora Weeks and Victor Bullen are a most important part of the history of the work, for without them the Back Remedies would surely not have survived. This book is a tribute to Nora and Victor, and their story is a delight to read.

Audio Cassette – Getting to know the Back Flower Remedies
Describing each Remedy, with exercises to assist the learner.

Video – The Light that Never Goes Out; the Story of the
Bach Flower Remedies
Dr Bach's life story and how his work continued from his home at Mount Vermont.

Pictorial Reference Cards

Illustrated in colour with descriptions and information concerning each Remedy.

The Bach Centre Newsletter

This is issued by the Bach Centre, Sotwell, and is published three times each year. It is an excellent way of keeping in touch and learning more.